THE LOW-FAT, HIGH-FIBER MACROBIOTICS DIET COOKBOOK

Enjoy Healthy, Nourishing Recipes to Beat Cancer, Lose Weight, Improve Digestion, and Maintain a Strong, Healthy Heart

Joe Miller, RD

Copyright Page

Table of Contents

Copyright Page 2

Table of Contents 3

Introduction to the Macrobiotic Diet 1

   Principles and Core Concepts 7

   Understanding Yin and Yang in Food 10

Macrobiotic Foods and Ingredients 15

   Other Macrobiotic Ingredients and Condiments

.... 17

   What Not to Eat on the Macrobiotic Diet 18

Cooking and Meal Preparation in Macrobiotics . 20

   Sample Macrobiotic Recipes 20

   Tips for Balancing Meals 25

   Seasonality and Locality in Food Selection 27

LOW-FAT, HIGH-FIBER MACROBIOTICS RECIPES FOR BREAKFAST 31

Flatbread with Avocado and Scallion Salsa 31

Green Energy 36

Cardamom Ambrosia Salad with Blue Cheese Dressing 39

Muesli Toast with Labneh, Hazelnuts, and Honey 42

The B.L.A. — Bagel with Lox and Avocado......43

Delicious Avocado Toast....................................44

Farmer's Wife's Breakfast..................................46

Greens and Grains Scramble 49

Super Energy Smoothie......................................52

Macrobiotic Grain Bowl 53

Miso Soup..55

Macrobiotic Sushi Rolls 56

Macrobiotic Buddha Bowl 58

Macrobiotic Stir-Fry 59

Macrobiotic Lentil Soup 61

LOW-FAT, HIGH-FIBER MACROBIOTICS RECIPES FOR LUNCH 64

Ricotta, broccoli & lemon penne 64

Spicy avocado wraps 66

Bean & feta spread with Greek salad salsa & oatcakes 68

Veggie meatballs with tomato courgetti 70

Moroccan spiced cauliflower & almond soup 73

Kale soup 74

Spinach & barley risotto 77

Cucumber, pea & lettuce soup 79

Mint & basil griddled peach salad 81

Courgette, pea & pesto soup 83

Cumin-spiced halloumi with corn & tomato slaw 85

Three bean salad with mozzarella 88

Black bean soup with chunky raita 91

Feta & clementine lunch bowl 94

Asparagus & lemon spaghetti with peas 96

LOW-FAT, HIGH-FIBER MACROBIOTICS RECIPES FOR DINNER 98

Soba noodle & edamame salad with grilled tofu 98

Green bean & penne salad with tomato and olive dressing 100

Delicious End-of-the-week veggie noodles with ginger & tamari...103

Quinoa with stir-fried winter veg..................105

Vegan paella 107

Moroccan-style vegetable platter 109

Vegan biryani 112

Sticky noodles with homemade hoisin 115

Penne with cabbage & walnuts 119

Courgette curry with lemon rice 121

Mint & basil griddled peach salad 125

Black bean chilli 127

Lentil ragu with courgetti 129

Chickpea, tomato & spinach curry 132

Noodle salad with sesame dressing 134

LOW-FAT, HIGH-FIBER MACROBIOTICS
RECIPES FOR BREAKFAST 138

Carrot & pecan muffins 138

Instant berry banana slush 140

Crispy roasted chickpeas 141

Date & buckwheat granola with pecans & seeds 143

Energy balls with dates 146

Avocado with tamari & ginger dressing 147

Polenta bruschetta with tapenade 148

Quinoa porridge 150

Vegetarian club...................153

Quinoa, peach & ginger bircher.....................154

Avocado & strawberry ices...................156

Masala omelette muffins 158

Red lentil & sweet potato pâté 160

Bean & feta spread with Greek salad salsa & oatcakes...................162

Melon & crunchy bran pots 164

LOW-FAT, HIGH-FIBER MACROBIOTICS RECIPES FOR BREAKFAST 166

Vegan kimchi 166

Chickpea, tomato & spinach curry 170

Red lentil & sweet potato pâté 172

Griddled vegetables with melting aubergines
....174

Barbecue sesame sweet potatoes......................177

Seeded soda bread..179

Red cabbage with apples....................................181

Pickled red cabbage 183

Spiced apple crisps...185

Summer sautéed potatoes 186

Thai carrot & radish salad.................................188

Red cabbage with mulled Port & pears 190

Carrot & sugar snap salad 192

Health Benefits and Considerations...................194

CHAPTER 1
Introduction to the Macrobiotic Diet

The macrobiotic diet has been around for hundreds of years and started as a way to eat that focused on nutrient-dense, seasonal foods harvested locally. This diet also focuses on balancing life, restorative exercise, and the elimination of any chemicals or artificial ingredients in both food and personal health products. Since coming to the United States in the 1970s, the diet has become a bit of a fad, both for good and not so good reasons.

Basics of the Macrobiotic Diet

The macrobiotic diet has been around since the 4th century BC, started as a concept in ancient Greece by the philosopher Hippocrates. It was then, as it mainly is today, a way of eating seasonal, local foods, mainly plants, exercising outside, sleeping well, and balancing life to the best of one's ability. Prussian physician Dr. Christoph Wilhelm Hufelan was the next to reintroduce the macrobiotic diet in 1796 with his book, Macrobiotics: The Art of Prolonging Life.

Again this concept faded away until the mid 19th century when, in Japan, Dr. Sagan Ishizuka started incorporating the macrobiotic diet principles into his own practice, which had relied heavily on Western medicine. Ishizuka had witnessed poor health among his army patients who weren't eating well, so he implemented a diet based on unrefined, whole, and fresh seasonal foods, cutting out any artificial ingredients, dairy and non-fish protein. The menu included foods such as whole grains, sea veggies, beans, locally grown and seasonal produce, nuts, seeds, and the occasional fish.

Like the other doctors before him, once Ishizuka died his practice faded away, and once again the macrobiotic diet was somewhat forgotten. That is until the 1920s when George Ohsawa, who was dying of tuberculosis, found Ishizuka's research and decided to try the macrobiotic diet himself. The results were extraordinary and Ohsawa made a full recovery. Ohsawa, along with his wife Lima, started teaching the philosophy and principles behind the macrobiotic diet, and eventually, the concept grew from Japan to Europe, and then all over the world. The macrobiotic diet was well received in the United States thanks to Michio Kushi, a student of Ohsawa and the founder of Erewhon Natural Foods, who popularized it in the 1970s.

The macrobiotic diet has changed over the centuries, and become more of a diet fad and lifestyle. It revolves around three main food principles including: Yin and yang

Macrobiotics emphasizes locally grown whole grain cereals, pulses (legumes), vegetables, edible seaweed, fermented soy products, and fruit combined into meals according to the ancient Chinese principle of balance known as yin and yang. Whole grains and whole-grain products such as brown rice and buckwheat pasta (soba), a variety of cooked and raw vegetables, beans and bean products, mild natural seasonings, fish, nuts and seeds, mild (non-stimulating) beverages such as bancha twig tea, and fruit are recommended.

Some macrobiotic proponents stress that yin and yang are relative qualities that can only be determined in a comparison. All food is considered to have both properties, with one dominating. Foods with yang qualities are considered compact, dense, heavy, and hot, whereas those with yin qualities are considered expansive, light, cold, and diffuse. However, these terms are relative; "yangness" or "yinness" is only discussed in relation to other foods.

Brown rice and other whole grains such as barley, millet, oats, quinoa, spelt, rye, and teff are considered by macrobiotics to be the foods in which yin and yang are closest to being in balance. Therefore, lists of macrobiotic foods that determine a food as yin or yang generally compare them to whole grains.

Nightshade vegetables, including tomatoes, peppers, potatoes, and eggplant; also, spinach, beets, and avocados, are not recommended or are used sparingly in macrobiotic cooking, as they are considered extremely yin. Some macrobiotic practitioners also discourage the use of nightshades because of the alkaloid solanine which is thought to affect calcium balance. Some proponents of a macrobiotic diet believe that nightshade vegetables can cause inflammation and osteoporosis.

The second is acid and alkaline, meaning one should consume foods with a high pH balance in order to create an alkaline-forming diet; finally, harmony with nature, one of the main reasons the macrobiotic diet is plant-based. This diet also follows the principles of loving life and following the five elements — fire, wood, water, metal, and earth — though these don't relate to the food as much as they do the lifestyle of the macrobiotic diet.

Principles and Core Concepts

The Japanese-style macrobiotic diet is founded on principles of balance and harmony, reflecting traditional Japanese dietary practices. Here's an elaboration on the guidelines outlined:

1. **Whole Cereal Grains**: The cornerstone of this diet, whole grains like brown rice form a significant portion, ranging from 40% to 60% of the daily intake. These grains are recommended to be chewed well, aiding in digestion and nutrient absorption.

2. **Vegetables**: Comprising 25% to 30% of the diet, vegetables provide essential vitamins, minerals, and fiber. They are versatile and can be consumed in various forms, including raw, steamed, or stir-fried.

3. **Beans and Legumes**: Making up about 5% to 10% of the diet, beans and legumes are excellent sources of protein, fiber, and essential nutrients. They are often included in soups, stews, or as side dishes.

4. **Miso Soup**: A staple in Japanese cuisine, miso soup contributes around 5% of the diet. Made from fermented soybeans, miso soup is rich in probiotics and adds flavor to meals.

5. **Sea Vegetables**: Also known as seaweed, sea vegetables provide minerals like iodine and calcium and are consumed in small amounts,

around 5% of the diet. They are often incorporated into salads, soups, or used as wraps.

6. **Traditionally or Naturally Processed Foods**: This category accounts for 5% to 10% of the diet and includes foods that are minimally processed or prepared using traditional methods, preserving their nutritional value.

Additionally, the diet allows for occasional consumption of fish and seafood, seeds and nuts, seed and nut butters, seasonings, sweeteners, fruits, and beverages, typically enjoyed two to three times per week. Natural animal products may also be included if necessary during dietary transitions or based on individual needs.

Regarding kitchenware, the emphasis is on using certain materials like wood or glass for cooking utensils, while avoiding materials such as plastic, copper, and non-stick coatings. Electric ovens are discouraged, likely due to concerns about potential chemical emissions during cooking.

Overall, the Japanese-style macrobiotic diet emphasizes whole, unprocessed foods, mindful eating practices, and harmony with nature, reflecting traditional Japanese values of balance and well-being.

Understanding Yin and Yang in Food

Yin & Yang Food

Yin and Yang is at the very heart of Feng Shui and Chinese philosophy. It is the essence of nature, where everything is in a perpetual state of change, moving from one extreme to the other to create equilibrium or universal balance.

The principles of Yin and Yang can also be applied to diet, and the term yin or yang relates to whether a food is a "cooling" or a "warming" food. However, these terms often have nothing to do with how it tastes or the way in which it is cooked, instead relating to the food's deeper essence. You might assume that all drinks are cooling; however beer is a cooling drink, but brandy is a warming drink.

Yang foods are warmer, drier and increase the internal heat of the body. Yin foods tend to cool, add moisture, and decrease the body's overall temperature. Yang foods also are also likely to contain more fat and provide the body with higher energy levels. Conversely, yin foods tend to have less fat but a higher water content.

Generally, a healthy, well-balanced meal should ideally consist of three parts yang and two parts yin foods. Using more yin foods than yang can also be helpful in calming children who tend to be hyperactive, but common sense must prevail and you should always seek medical advice before making major changes to any diet.

Foods fall into three categories;

• Yin foods

• Yang foods

• Neutral foods

Here is a very basic food list.

Yin Food

Almonds, Apple, Asparagus, Bamboo, Banana, Barley, Bean curd, Bean sprouts, Beer, Broccoli, Cabbage, Celery, Clams, Corn, Corn flour, Crab, Cucumber, Duck, Eel, Fish, Grapes, Honey, Ice creams, Lemons, Mushrooms, Mussels, Oranges, Oysters, Peppermint tea, Pineapple, Salt, Shrimps, Spinach, Strawberries, Soya beans, White sugar, Tomatoes, Water.

Yang Food

Beef, Black pepper, Brown sugar, Butter, Cheese, Chicken liver, skin, and fat, Chillies, Chocolate, Coffee, Eggs, Fish (smoked), Garlic, Green peppers, Goose, Ham, Kidney beans, Lamb, Leeks, Onions, Peanut butter, Roasted peanuts, Pork, Potato, Rabbit, Turkey, Walnuts, Whisky, Wine.

Neutral Food

Bread, Carrots, Cauliflower, Cherries, Lean chicken meat, Dates, Figs, Milk, Olives, Peaches, Peas, Pigeon, Plums, Pork, Raisins, Brown rice, Steamed white rice, Sweet Potato.

The main crux of the macrobiotic diet is whole grains, and many meals contain around 50-percent of this food. This includes

- bulgur wheat

- buckwheat

- brown rice

- quinoa

- wild rice

Whole cereal grains are considered preferable to whole-grain pastas and breads. That said, these types of processed food are permissible in small quantities.

Fresh Vegetables

Fresh, seasonal, and locally sourced vegetables are another major part of the diet, especially leafy greens like kale, bok choy, and chard. This part makes up about 30-percent of the daily food intake, and vegetables can be steamed, boiled, sautéed, or baked. There are some who follow the diet that recommend avoiding nightshades such as potatoes, tomatoes, eggplant, and peppers, as well as beets, summer squash, and spinach, but these foods are not rigorously prohibited. However non-local fruit is highly discouraged.

Protein

A bit of fresh seafood or fish for protein is allowed, though it's not usually eaten every day. Mostly the protein in the macrobiotic diet comes from beans, especially soybeans. While processed food, in general, isn't part of the diet, soybeans made into tofu, bean curd, or tempeh are allowed. Soy also comes into play in miso form, namely as a soup. A broth-based soup, in fact, is to be eaten twice a day, every day. Lightly roasted and salted nuts and/or seeds too can be added, but no more than one ounce every few days.

Other Macrobiotic Ingredients and Condiments

Oils and Spices: To cook foods, avoid olive or coconut oil. Instead, the approved types of cooking oils for the macrobiotic diet include light or dark sesame oil, unrefined vegetable oil, corn oil, or mustard seed oil. Spices can be used and often the macrobiotic diet features Japanese condiments and flavorings such as fermented pickles, shoyu, grated ginger, brown rice and umeboshi vinegars, umeboshi plums, and roasted seaweed.

What Not to Eat on the Macrobiotic Diet

The main thing to remember when cooking for or following a macrobiotic diet is to eschew chemicals, processed food, dairy, and non-fish meat. The list of banned foods also includes eggs, refined sugar, honey, molasses, coffee, black tea, and alcohol. Once those are eliminated, cooking for the macrobiotic diet doesn't prove difficult. More, it's challenging to plan, and takes effort to prepare the right foods for each meal of the day.

CHAPTER 3
Cooking and Meal Preparation in
Macrobiotics

The main methods of cooking on the macrobiotic diet include steaming, sautéeing, eating raw, boiled, and baking. The main thing to think about when cooking for this diet is what is being prepared.

Sample Macrobiotic Recipes

1. **Macrobiotic Brown Rice Congee**: Congee is a traditional Asian rice porridge known for its digestibility and soothing qualities. In this macrobiotic version, brown rice is simmered with plenty of water until it reaches a creamy texture.

It's delicious plain or topped with scallions, shredded nori, and a drizzle of sesame oil.

2. **Macrobiotic Vegetable Stir-Fry**: This recipe combines seasonal vegetables sautéed in a bit of sesame oil or tamari. Common veggies include cabbage, carrots, kale, bell peppers, and mushrooms. Serve over brown rice or quinoa for a satisfying meal.

3. **Macrobiotic Noodle Soup**: A comforting noodle soup made with whole grain noodles, miso broth, and an array of vegetables. Customize it with tofu, seaweed, or green onions. Perfect for chilly days.

4. **Macrobiotic Hijiki Salad**: Hijiki, a type of seaweed, stars in this salad. Soak dried hijiki until rehydrated, then mix with grated carrots, tofu cubes, and a dressing of tamari, sesame oil, and rice vinegar. It's a nutritious and flavorful side dish.

5. **Macrobiotic Azuki Bean Stew**: Azuki beans are a staple in macrobiotic cuisine for their nourishing qualities. Simmer them with squash, sweet potatoes, and onions in a flavorful broth. Season with ginger, garlic, and tamari for depth of flavor.

6. **Macrobiotic Sushi Rolls**: Make sushi rolls macrobiotic-friendly by using brown rice and filling them with veggies like cucumber, avocado,

and pickled radish. Serve with tamari and wasabi for dipping.

7. **Macrobiotic Pumpkin Soup**: Creamy soup made from roasted pumpkin, onions, garlic, and vegetable broth. Season with warming spices like ginger, cinnamon, and nutmeg for a cozy meal.

8. **Macrobiotic Millet Porridge**: Millet, a nutritious whole grain, forms the base of this porridge. Customize it sweet with almond milk, cinnamon, and chopped fruits, or savory with sautéed greens and nutritional yeast.

These recipes highlight the diversity and creativity of macrobiotic cooking, focusing on whole grains, seasonal veggies, legumes, and seaweed for a balanced and nourishing diet.

Tips for Balancing Meals

1. Start your meals with hearty servings of whole grains like brown rice, barley, or quinoa. These provide essential carbs, fiber, and nutrients to fuel your day.

2. Incorporate beans and legumes such as lentils and chickpeas for a satisfying dose of plant-based protein and fiber. They're nutritious and versatile, perfect for adding depth to your meals.

3. Fill your plate with a diverse array of locally sourced, seasonal vegetables. Think dark leafy greens, vibrant root veggies, and nutrient-packed seaweed to ensure a well-rounded nutritional profile.

4. Sea veggies like nori and wakame are not only flavorful but also packed with essential minerals

like iodine. Sprinkle them into your dishes for a nutritional boost and a taste of the ocean.

5. While fat intake is generally low in a macrobiotic diet, incorporating small amounts of healthy fats from sources like sesame oil, seeds, and nuts can provide essential fatty acids and enhance flavor.

6. Limit animal products, opting for small portions of fish like sardines or mackerel for omega-3 fatty acids if desired. Plant-based proteins should take center stage in your meals.

7. Prioritize seasonal and locally grown produce for optimal freshness and flavor. Not only does this support local farmers, but it also ensures you're getting the best-quality ingredients available.

8. Take your time to savor each bite, chewing thoroughly and enjoying the flavors and textures

of your food. Being mindful of portion sizes and listening to your body's hunger cues helps maintain balance.

9. Aim for a balance of yin and yang foods in your meals, incorporating a mix of expansive and contractive elements for overall harmony and well-being.

10. Don't forget to drink plenty of water throughout the day to stay hydrated and support your body's natural functions.

Seasonality and Locality in Food Selection

In a macrobiotic diet, emphasizing seasonal and local foods is crucial for maximizing freshness and flavor while aligning with the principles of balance and harmony for the following reasons:

1. **Nutritional Abundance**: Seasonal foods are typically harvested at their peak ripeness, containing higher levels of nutrients compared to off-season counterparts. Consuming foods when they're in season maximizes their nutritional benefits.

2. **Environmental Sustainability**: Choosing locally grown foods reduces the carbon footprint associated with transportation and storage. Supporting local farmers promotes sustainable agricultural practices and helps preserve the environment.

3. **Connection to Nature**: Eating with the seasons fosters a deeper connection to nature and the

Earth's cycles. It encourages mindfulness and appreciation for the natural abundance available throughout the year and further emphasizes the principles of harmony.

4. **Variety and Diversity**: Seasonal eating encourages a varied diet as different fruits, vegetables, and grains come into season at different times. This variety ensures a broader spectrum of nutrients and flavors in meals.

5. **Harmony with Climate and Body**: Consuming foods in harmony with the local climate and environment is believed to promote balance within the body according to traditional Chinese medicine and macrobiotic philosophy. For instance, cooling foods like cucumbers are more prevalent in the summer, while hearty root vegetables are favored in colder months.

6. **Taste and Quality**: Seasonal foods often taste better due to their freshness and minimal storage or transportation. Enjoying produce at its peak ensures optimal flavor and quality.

When selecting foods for a macrobiotic diet, consider what's in season in your region and aim to source ingredients locally whenever possible. This approach enhances the nutritional value of meals and contributes to a more sustainable and harmonious lifestyle.

Flatbread with Avocado and Scallion Salsa

Ingredients

8 servings

Dough:

1 ½ tsp. sugar

1 (¼-oz.) envelope active dry yeast (about 2¼ tsp.)

2½ cups (313 g) all-purpose flour

½ cup whole-milk plain Greek yogurt

2 Tbsp. extra-virgin olive oil

2 tsp. kosher salt

Salsa and assembly:

2 tsp. coriander seeds

2 tsp. cumin seeds

8 scallions

4 Tbsp. plus 1 cup extra-virgin olive oil, divided, plus more for brushing

Kosher salt

1 red or green chile (such as serrano or jalapeño), finely chopped

1 cup finely chopped parsley

1 lemon

4 medium avocados, pits removed

Flaky sea salt (optional)

Special Equipment: A spice mill

Preparation

Dough:

Step 1

Stir sugar into ¾ cup warm water in a large bowl. Sprinkle in yeast and let sit until foamy, about 10 minutes.

Step 2

Add flour, yogurt, oil, and kosher salt to sugar mixture and mix until a shaggy dough forms (don't worry about any dry or unincorporated bits). Cover bowl with a damp kitchen towel and let sit in a warm, dry spot until doubled in size, about 1 hour.

Salsa and assembly:

Step 3

While the dough is rising, toast coriander seeds and cumin seeds in a dry medium skillet over medium heat, shaking often, until fragrant and slightly darkened in color, about 3 minutes. Transfer to a spice mill. Let cool, then coarsely grind. Set spice mixture aside.

Step 4

Place scallions and 1 Tbsp. oil in skillet, season with kosher salt, and cook, turning occasionally, until softened and deeply charred, about 4 minutes. Transfer to a cutting board; trim roots and discard. Finely chop scallions and place in a medium bowl. Add reserved spice mixture, chile, and parsley. Finely grate half of lemon zest into bowl, then cut lemon in half and squeeze in juice.

Add 1 cup oil and stir well to combine. Season with kosher salt and let sit while you make the flatbreads.

Step 5

Turn out dough onto a lightly dusted surface and divide into 8 equal pieces. Form into balls and, working with 1 ball at a time, roll out into 6" rounds about ¼" thick.

Step 6

Heat 1 Tbsp. oil in a large skillet over medium-high. Working 1 at a time and adding remaining 2 Tbsp. oil as needed, cook flatbread until bubbles appear over the surface, about 1 minute. Flip and cook until cooked through, about 1 minute. Continue to cook, turning often, until browned in spots on both sides, about 1 minute longer.

Transfer to a plate and wrap up in a clean kitchen towel to keep warm.

Step 7

To serve, brush each flatbread with oil. Coarsely smash avocados onto flatbread and spoon salsa over. Sprinkle with sea salt if desired.

Green Energy

Ingredients

Serves 1

1 pear, halved

1/4 cucumber, roughly chopped

1 1/2 cups young spinach

4 sprigs of fresh flat-leaf parsley

1/2 avocado, pitted and flesh scooped from the skin

1/2 teaspoon spirulina powder

chilled water, to taste

1 brazil nut, coarsely chopped

Preparation

Mix it up

Feed the pear and cucumber through a juicer. Pour the juice into a blender, add the spinach, parsley, and avocado, and blend until smooth. Pour into a glass. Mix the spirulina with just enough water to make a thick liquid, then swirl it into the juice. Sprinkle with the chopped brazil nut, then serve.

Cardamom Ambrosia Salad with Blue Cheese Dressing

Ingredients

For the dressing:

2 1/2 ounces blue cheese

3 tablespoons buttermilk

3 tablespoons sour cream

2 teaspoons white wine vinegar

1/4 teaspoon sugar

Salt and freshly ground black pepper to taste

For the salad:

2 oranges, cut into suprêmes

1 grapefruit, cut into suprêmes

2 Champagne mangoes, peeled, pitted, and thinly sliced

2 Anjou pears, cored and thinly sliced

1/2 cup shredded fresh coconut

3 ounces pitted dates, coarsely chopped, plus more for garnish

1/4 cup slivered almonds

3/4 teaspoon ground cardamom

2 teaspoons coconut water

Chopped fresh flat-leaf parsley, for garnish

Preparation

Make the dressing:

Step 1

Mash the cheese in a small bowl with a fork. Add the remaining Ingredients and whisk until combined but still a bit lumpy.

Make the salad:

Step 2

Combine the orange, grapefruit, mango, and pear slices in a medium bowl. Add the shredded coconut, dates, and almonds, then sprinkle with the cardamom, add the coconut water, and thoroughly toss the salad. Add the dressing and toss together.

Step 3

Divided the salad among individual bowls or serve it in a large bowl for a family-style dinner.

Garnish with more chopped dates and some parsley, if desired.

Muesli Toast with Labneh, Hazelnuts, and Honey

Ingredients

Servings

Hazelnuts

Olive oil

Salt and pepper

Seeded bread

Labneh or Greek yogurt

Honey

Preparation

Toss chopped toasted hazelnuts in a little olive oil; season with salt and pepper. Spread toasted thin seeded bread with labneh or Greek yogurt. Top with hazelnuts and drizzle with honey.

The B.L.A. — Bagel with Lox and Avocado

Ingredients

Makes 2 servings

1 small ripe avocado, preferably Hass (see Note)

1 teaspoon fresh lemon juice, or to taste

Salt and freshly ground black pepper

2 bagels

2 slices or 4 thin strips of lox, or smoked salmon

2 thin slices of red onion

4 thin slices of tomato

1 teaspoon capers, rinsed (optional)

Preparation

A short time before serving, mash avocado and add lemon juice. Season with pepper and only a bit of salt, as there will be enough in the lox. Split bagels and spread each half with avocado. Top with lox. Put onion, tomato, and capers (if using) on bottom half, then set top half of sandwich in place. Serve at once.

Delicious Avocado Toast

Ingredients

Servings

Cucumber

Fresh lime juice

Crushed red pepper flakes

Salt and pepper

Sourdough bread

Tahini

Avocado

Olive oil

Preparation

Season thinly sliced cucumber with fresh lime juice, crushed red pepper flakes, salt, and pepper. Spread toasted sourdough bread with tahini and top with smashed avocado; season with salt and pepper. Top with cucumber and a drizzle of olive oil.

Farmer's Wife's Breakfast

Ingredients

2 servings with leftover patties

Lamb sausage patties:

1 pound ground lamb

2 tablespoons ground fennel seed

2 tablespoons apple cider vinegar

2 tablespoons coconut aminos

1 teaspoon smoked sea salt

1 tablespoon ghee, divided

Salad:

2 handfuls of greens such as arugula, mizuna, baby kale, or baby spinach

2 tablespoons extra virgin olive oil

1 tablespoon freshly squeezed lemon juice

Dash of sea salt

Sides:

1 ripe avocado, peeled, pitted, and sliced

1 cup store- bought sauerkraut

1/2 cup fresh pomegranate seeds

Preparation

Step 1

To make the patties, in a large bowl, knead together the lamb, fennel seed, apple cider vinegar, coconut aminos, and salt. Using your hands, form the mixture into twelve patties.

Step 2

In a skillet over medium- high heat, heat 1 1/2 teaspoons ghee. Place six patties in the hot skillet and fry for 4 minutes or until brown. Flip and fry for 3 minutes. Set aside. Add the remaining ghee to the skillet and fry the remaining patties.

Step 3

To make the salad, in a medium bowl, toss the greens with the olive oil, lemon, and salt until well coated. To serve, place half the salad on each plate and top with two patties and half the avocado, sauerkraut, and pomegranate seeds. Store the remaining patties for the next day's breakfast.

Greens and Grains Scramble

Ingredients

Serves 2, heartily

4 large eggs, beaten

1 tablespoon milk

1/4 teaspoon kosher salt

2 tablespoons extra-virgin olive oil

1 green onion, white and light green parts, finely chopped (about 1 tablespoon)

2 cloves garlic, minced

1 heaping cup / 240 ml well-packed chopped leafy greens (such as kale, Swiss chard leaves without ribs, or spinach)

1/2 cup / 120 ml cooked whole grains (wheat berries, farro, barley, or millet)

1 tablespoon chopped fresh chives

Freshly ground black pepper

Flaky salt

Crusty bread, toasted English muffins, or warm corn tortillas, for serving

Preparation

Step 1

In a large bowl, whisk together the eggs, milk, and kosher salt; set aside. Heat 1 tablespoon of the olive oil in a sauté pan over medium heat. Add the green onion and garlic and sauté until soft, 1 to 2 minutes. Add the greens, grains, and remaining 1 tablespoon olive oil and sauté until the greens are wilted and the grains are warmed through, 3 to 5 minutes.

Step 2

Decrease the heat to low and pour in the egg mixture, gently stirring to comingle them with the greens and grains. Continue stirring until they're softly scrambled, 2 to 3 minutes. Remove from the heat, stir in the chives, and season with pepper.

Step 3

Serve hot with a sprinkling of flaky salt on top, and crusty bread, toasted English muffins, or warm corn tortillas alongside.

Super Energy Smoothie

Ingredients

Makes 2 servings

1 cup vanilla soymilk

1 cup firm light tofu (about 6 oz)

3/4 cup fresh blueberries (or 1/2 cup frozen, unsweetened)

2 scoops soy-protein powder (1 scoop is about 3 tbsp)

1 tsp almond extract

Preparation

Place all Ingredients in blender and mix on high until smooth and creamy.

Macrobiotic Grain Bowl

Ingredients

- 1 cup cooked brown rice

- 1 cup steamed kale

- 1/2 cup cooked chickpeas

- 1/4 cup shredded carrots

- 1/4 cup sliced cucumber

- 1 tablespoon sesame seeds

- 2 tablespoons tamari sauce

- 1 tablespoon rice vinegar

- 1 teaspoon grated ginger

Preparation

1. In a bowl, arrange cooked brown rice as the base.

2. Top with steamed kale, cooked chickpeas, shredded carrots, and sliced cucumber.

3. In a separate small bowl, mix tamari sauce, rice vinegar, and grated ginger to make the dressing.

4. Drizzle the dressing over the bowl and sprinkle sesame seeds on top.

5. Serve and enjoy!

Miso Soup

Ingredients

- 4 cups water

- 2 tablespoons miso paste

- 1/2 cup diced tofu

- 1/4 cup sliced green onions

- 1/2 cup sliced mushrooms

- 1 sheet nori (seaweed), torn into small pieces

- 1 tablespoon tamari sauce

Preparation

1. In a pot, bring water to a simmer.

2. Dissolve miso paste in a small amount of water and add it to the pot.

3. Add tofu, green onions, mushrooms, nori, and tamari sauce to the pot.

4. Simmer for 5-10 minutes until heated through.

5. Serve hot and enjoy!

Macrobiotic Sushi Rolls

Ingredients

- Nori sheets

- Cooked brown rice

- Assorted vegetables (carrots, cucumber, avocado, bell peppers)

- Tamari sauce

- Pickled ginger

- Wasabi (optional)

Preparation

1. Place a nori sheet on a sushi mat.

2. Spread a thin layer of cooked brown rice over the nori sheet.

3. Arrange sliced vegetables in the center of the rice.

4. Roll the nori sheet tightly using the sushi mat.

5. Slice the roll into bite-sized pieces.

6. Serve with tamari sauce, pickled ginger, and wasabi.

7. Enjoy your homemade macrobiotic sushi rolls!

Macrobiotic Buddha Bowl

Ingredients

- Cooked quinoa or millet

- Steamed broccoli

- Sautéed tofu or tempeh

- Sliced radishes

- Shredded cabbage

- Sprouts (alfalfa, mung bean, or broccoli sprouts)

- Tahini dressing (tahini, lemon juice, water, salt)

Preparation

1. Arrange cooked quinoa or millet as the base of the bowl.

2. Top with steamed broccoli, sautéed tofu or tempeh, sliced radishes, shredded cabbage, and sprouts.

3. Drizzle with tahini dressing.

4. Serve and enjoy the nutritious Buddha bowl!

Macrobiotic Stir-Fry

Ingredients

- Assorted vegetables (broccoli, bell peppers, carrots, snap peas)

- Firm tofu, cubed

- 2 tablespoons tamari sauce

- 1 tablespoon sesame oil

- 1 garlic clove, minced

- 1 teaspoon grated ginger

- Cooked brown rice or soba noodles

Preparation

1. Heat sesame oil in a skillet over medium heat.

2. Add minced garlic and grated ginger, sauté for a minute.

3. Add cubed tofu to the skillet and cook until lightly browned.

4. Add assorted vegetables and tamari sauce to the skillet.

5. Stir-fry until vegetables are tender-crisp.

6. Serve over cooked brown rice or soba noodles.

7. Enjoy your flavorful macrobiotic stir-fry!

Macrobiotic Lentil Soup

Ingredients

- 1 cup dried lentils

- 4 cups vegetable broth

- 1 onion, diced

- 2 carrots, diced

- 2 celery stalks, diced

- 2 garlic cloves, minced

- 1 tablespoon olive oil

- 1 teaspoon ground cumin

- 1 teaspoon dried thyme

- Salt and pepper to taste

- Fresh parsley for garnish

Preparation

1. Heat olive oil in a pot over medium heat.

2. Add diced onion, carrots, and celery, sauté until softened.

3. Add minced garlic, ground cumin, and dried thyme, sauté for another minute.

4. Add dried lentils and vegetable broth to the pot.

5. Bring to a boil, then reduce heat and simmer for about 20-25 minutes until lentils are tender.

6. Season with salt and pepper to taste.

7. Serve hot, garnished with fresh parsley.

8. Enjoy.

Ricotta, broccoli & lemon penne

Ingredients

200g wholemeal penne

1 leek, washed and sliced

200g broccoli, cut into small florets

1 tbsp rapeseed oil

1 red pepper, deseeded, quartered and sliced

1 tsp finely chopped rosemary

1 red chilli, deseeded and sliced

3 garlic cloves, sliced

1 lemon, zested and juiced

3 tbsp ricotta

Preparations

STEP 1

Boil the pasta with the leeks for 7 mins, then add the broccoli and boil for 5 mins more until just tender.

STEP 2

Meanwhile, heat the oil and fry the pepper with the rosemary, chilli and garlic in a large non-stick pan for 5 mins until softened.

STEP 3

Drain the pasta and veg, reserving a little water, then tip the pasta and veg into the pan. Add the lemon zest and juice, ricotta, and some pasta water. Pile into bowls.

Spicy avocado wraps

Ingredients

0.5 x 300g pack mycoprotein chicken-style pieces (or similar vegetarian product), sliced at an angle

generous squeeze juice 0.5 lime

½ tsp mild chilli powder

1 garlic clove, chopped

1 tsp olive oil

2 seeded wraps

1 avocado, halved and stoned

1 roasted red pepper, from a jar

few sprigs coriander, chopped

Preparations

STEP 1

Mix the vegetarian, chicken-style pieces with the lime juice, chilli powder and garlic.

STEP 2

Heat the oil in a non-stick frying pan then fry the pieces for a couple of mins, while you warm the wraps following the pack instructions or if you have a gas hob, heat them over the flame to slightly char them. Do not let them dry out or they are difficult to roll.

STEP 3

Squash half an avocado onto each wrap, add the peppers to the pan to warm them through then pile onto the wraps with the chicken-style pieces, and sprinkle over the coriander. Roll up, cut in half and eat with your fingers.

Bean & feta spread with Greek salad salsa & oatcakes

Ingredients

400g can butter beans, drained

1 lemon, ½ juiced, ½ cut into 4 wedges

2 tbsp ricotta or bio yogurt

85g feta, crumbled

1 garlic clove

12 oatcakes

For the salsa

4 tomatoes, chopped

1 medium cucumber, finely diced

1 small red onion, finely chopped

12 pitted Kalamata olives, chopped

A few chopped mint leaves (optional)

Preparations

STEP 1

Tip the beans, lemon juice, ricotta, 50g feta and the garlic into a bowl and blitz with a hand blender or in a food processor to make a paste. Stir in the remaining feta and spoon the mixture into four small pots.

STEP 2

To make the salsa, stir all the Ingredients together with the mint (if using) and divide into four more pots, topping with a lemon wedge. These will keep, chilled in an airtight container, for two-three days. To eat, spread the oatcakes with the bean mixture, squeeze the lemon wedges over the salads and pile generously onto the oatcakes.

Veggie meatballs with tomato courgetti

Ingredients

3 garlic cloves

For the veggie meatballs

2 tsp rapeseed oil, plus extra for greasing

1 small onion, very finely chopped

2 tsp balsamic vinegar

100g canned red kidney beans

1 tbsp beaten egg

1 tsp tomato purée

1 heaped tsp chilli powder

½ tsp ground coriander

15g ground almonds

40g cooked sweetcorn

2 tsp chopped thyme leaves

For the tomato courgetti

2 large or 3 normal tomatoes, chopped

1 tsp tomato purée

1 tsp balsamic vinegar

2 courgettes cut into 'noodles' with a spiralizer, julienne peeler, or by hand

Preparations

STEP 1

Finely chop the garlic. Heat the oil in a large pan and fry the onion, stirring frequently, for 8 mins. Stir in the balsamic vinegar and cook for 2 mins more. Meanwhile, put the beans in a bowl with the egg, tomato purée and spices, and mash until smooth. Stir in the almonds and sweetcorn with the thyme, a third of the chopped garlic and the balsamic onions. Mix well and shape into about 8 balls the size of a walnut, and place on a baking tray lined with oiled baking parchment.

Moroccan spiced cauliflower & almond soup

Ingredients

1 large cauliflower

2 tbsp olive oil

½ tsp each ground cinnamon, cumin and coriander

2 tbsp harissa paste, plus extra drizzle

1l hot vegetable or chicken stock

50g toasted flaked almond, plus extra to serve

Preparations

STEP 1

Cut the cauliflower into small florets. Fry olive oil, ground cinnamon, cumin and coriander and harissa paste for 2 mins in a large pan. Add the cauliflower, stock and almonds. Cover and cook for 20 mins until the cauliflower is tender. Blend soup until smooth, then serve with an extra drizzle of harissa and a sprinkle of toasted almonds.

Kale soup

Ingredients

2 tbsp rapeseed oil

3 onions (320g), finely chopped

3 garlic cloves, finely grated

125g celery, chopped

2 yellow peppers, deseeded and diced

2 tsp smoked paprika

400g can chopped tomatoes

2 tsp dried oregano

1 litre hot vegetable stock, made with 3 tsp bouillon powder

150g wholemeal penne

200g green beans, trimmed and cut into short lengths

200g cavolo nero (kale), thinly sliced

160g cherry tomatoes

30g pack of basil, chopped

80g vegetarian Italian-style hard cheese, finely grated

Preparations

STEP 1

Heat the oil in a large pan over a medium heat and fry the onions and garlic for 5 mins, then add the celery and peppers. Fry for another 5 mins, adding the smoked paprika in the last minute. Stir in the tomatoes, oregano and stock. Bring to the boil.

STEP 2

Tip in the penne, green beans and kale, bring back to the boil and cook over a medium heat for 10 mins. Stir in the cherry tomatoes and basil, and cook for a few minutes more until the tomatoes have burst.

Spinach & barley risotto

Ingredients

2 tsp rapeseed oil

1 large leek (315g), thinly sliced

2 garlic cloves, chopped

2 x 400g can barley, undrained

1 tbsp vegetable bouillon powder

1 tsp finely chopped sage

1 tbsp thyme leaves

160g cherry tomatoes, halved

160g spinach

50g finely grated vegetarian Italian-style hard cheese

Preparations

STEP 1

Heat the oil in a non-stick pan and fry the leek and garlic for 5-10 mins, stirring frequently, until softened, adding a splash of water if it sticks.

STEP 2

Tip in the cans of barley and their liquid, then stir in the bouillon powder, sage and thyme. Simmer, stirring frequently, for 4-5 mins. Add the tomatoes and spinach and cook for 2-3 mins more until the spinach is wilted, adding a splash more water if needed. Stir in most of the cheese, then serve with the remaining cheese scattered over.

Cucumber, pea & lettuce soup

Ingredients

1 tsp rapeseed oil

small bunch spring onions, roughly chopped

1 cucumber, roughly chopped

1 large round lettuce, roughly chopped

225g frozen peas

4 tsp vegetable bouillon

4 tbsp bio yogurt (optional)

4 slices rye bread

Preparations

STEP 1

Boil 1.4 litres water in a kettle. Heat the oil in a large non-stick frying pan and cook the spring onions for 5 mins, stirring frequently, or until softened. Add the cucumber, lettuce and peas, then pour in the boiled water. Stir in the bouillon, cover and simmer for 10 mins or until the vegetables are soft but still bright green.

STEP 2

Blitz the mixture with a hand blender until smooth. Serve hot or cold, topped with yogurt (if you like), with rye bread alongside.

Mint & basil griddled peach salad

Ingredients

1 lime, zested and juiced

1 tbsp rapeseed oil

2 tbsp finely chopped mint, plus a few whole leaves to serve

2 tbsp basil, chopped

2 peaches (300g), quartered

75g quinoa

160g fine beans, trimmed and halved

1 small red onion, very finely chopped

1 large Little Gem lettuce (165g), roughly chopped

½ x 60g pack rocket

1 small avocado, stoned and sliced

Preparations

STEP 1

Mix the lime zest and juice, oil, mint and basil, then put half in a bowl with the peaches. Meanwhile, cook the quinoa following pack instructions.

STEP 2

Cook the beans for 3-4 mins until just tender. Meanwhile, griddle the peaches for 1 min on each side. If you don't have a griddle pan, use a large non-stick frying pan with a drop of oil.

STEP 3

Drain the quinoa and divide between shallow bowls. Toss the warm beans and onion in the remaining mint mixture and pile on top of the quinoa with the lettuce and rocket. Top with the avocado and peaches and scatter over the mint leaves. Serve while still warm.

Courgette, pea & pesto soup

Ingredients

1 tbsp olive oil

1 garlic clove, sliced

500g courgettes, quartered lengthways and chopped

200g frozen peas

400g can cannellini beans, drained and rinsed

1l hot vegetable stock

2 tbsp basil pesto, or vegetarian alternative

Preparations

STEP 1

Heat the oil in a large saucepan. Cook the garlic for a few seconds, then add the courgettes and cook for 3 mins until they start to soften. Stir in the peas and cannellini beans, pour on the hot stock and cook for a further 3 mins.

STEP 2

Stir the pesto through the soup with some seasoning, then ladle into bowls and serve with crusty brown bread, if you like. Or pop in a flask to take to work.

Cumin-spiced halloumi with corn & tomato slaw

Ingredients

1 lime, zested and juiced

1 tsp rapeseed oil

1 tsp fresh thyme leaves

¼ tsp turmeric

¼ tsp cumin seeds

1 tbsp finely chopped coriander

1 garlic clove, finely grated

100g halloumi, thinly sliced

For the slaw

1 lime, zested and juiced

3 tbsp bio yogurt

3 tbsp finely chopped coriander

1 red chilli, deseeded and chopped

160g corn, cut from 2 fresh cobs

1 red pepper, deseeded and chopped

100g fine green beans, blanched, trimmed and halved

200g cherry tomatoes, halved

1 red onion, halved and finely sliced

320g white cabbage, finely sliced

Preparations

STEP 1

Mix the lime zest and juice with the oil, thyme, turmeric, cumin, coriander and garlic together in a bowl. Add the halloumi and carefully turn it until coated – take care as it breaks easily.

STEP 2

To make the slaw, mix the lime juice and zest, yogurt, coriander and chilli together, then stir in the corn, red pepper, beans, tomatoes, onion and cabbage.

STEP 3

Heat a large non-stick frying pan or griddle pan and fry the cheese in batches for 1 min each side. Serve the slaw on plates with the halloumi slices on top. If you're cooking for two people, serve half of the halloumi and slaw and chill the rest for lunch another day.

Three bean salad with mozzarella

Ingredients

320g fine beans, ends trimmed and halved if large

4 carrots (320g), cut into slim batons

2 red onions, halved and sliced

400g can cannellini beans, drained

400g can red kidney beans, drained

320g mixed colour baby tomatoes (ours were red, yellow and orange), halved

15g basil leaves, roughly torn

120g vegetarian mozzarella, cut into cubes

For the dressing

2 tbsp extra virgin olive oil

1-2 tbsp balsamic vinegar

2 garlic cloves, finely chopped

½-1 tsp dried oregano

1 tsp dried English mustard powder

15 pitted Kalamata olives (about 45g), sliced

½ tsp lemon zest and 2 tbsp juice

Preparations

STEP 1

Boil or steam the green beans and carrots for 8-10 mins until just tender. Put the sliced onions in a bowl and pour over boiling water until just covered.

STEP 2

Meanwhile, make the dressing. Mix all the Ingredients together in a large bowl.

STEP 3

Tip the cooked beans and carrots into the dressing along with the drained onions, canned beans and tomatoes, toss well, then add the basil and toss again. Serve scattered with the mozzarella and a grinding of black pepper, if you like. Will keep chilled for up to three days.

Black bean soup with chunky raita

Ingredients

1-1½ tsp cumin seeds

2 tsp smoked paprika

2 tsp ground coriander

4 x 400g cans black beans

400g can chopped tomatoes

1 tbsp tomato purée

1 tbsp vegetable bouillon powder

3 large garlic cloves, finely grated

2 small avocados, chopped

For the raita

200g cherry tomatoes, quartered, smaller ones halved

2 spring onions, finely chopped

2 tbsp lemon juice

2 x 120g pots bio yogurt

15g coriander, chopped, plus extra to serve

Preparations

STEP 1

Toast the cumin seeds briefly in a large saucepan over a medium heat. Spoon in the paprika and coriander, then tip in 2½ cans of beans along with their liquid, the tomatoes, tomato purée, bouillon, garlic and 500ml water. Cover and leave to simmer for 15 mins.

STEP 2

Meanwhile, stir the Ingredients for the raita together in a bowl.

STEP 3

Blitz the cooked beans using a hand blender until completely smooth, then stir in the remaining beans and return to the boil. Serve half and top with half the raita, a chopped avocado and some extra coriander. Leave the remaining soup to cool, then chill for another day. Will keep chilled for four days; the raita will keep for two days. Reheat the soup in a pan over a low-medium heat until piping hot.

Feta & clementine lunch bowl

Ingredients

1 red onion, halved and thinly sliced

1 lemon, zested and juiced

2 clementines, 1 zested, flesh sliced

2 garlic cloves, chopped

400g can green lentils, drained

1 tbsp balsamic vinegar

1 ½ tbsp rapeseed oil

1 red pepper, quartered and sliced

60g feta, crumbled

small handful mint, chopped

4 walnut halves, chopped

Preparations

STEP 1

Mix the onion with the lemon juice, lemon and clementine zest and garlic.

STEP 2

Tip the lentils into two bowls or lunchboxes and drizzle over the balsamic and 1 tbsp oil. Heat the remaining oil in a large non-stick wok, add the pepper and stir-fry for 3 mins. Tip in half the onion and cook until tender. Pile on top of the lentils, then mix the clementines, remaining onions, feta, mint and walnut pieces.

Asparagus & lemon spaghetti with peas

Ingredients

150g wholemeal spaghetti

160g asparagus, ends trimmed and cut into lengths

2 tbsp rapeseed oil

2 leeks (220g), cut into lengths, then thin strips

1 red chilli, deseeded and finely chopped

1 garlic clove, finely grated

160g frozen peas

1 lemon, zested and juiced, plus wedges to serve

Preparations

STEP 1

Boil the spaghetti for 12 mins until al dente, adding the asparagus for the last 3 mins. Meanwhile, heat the oil in a large non-stick frying pan, add the leeks and chilli and cook for 5 mins. Stir in the garlic, peas and lemon zest and juice and cook for a few mins more.

STEP 2

Drain and add the pasta to the pan with ¼ mug of the pasta water and toss everything together until well mixed. Spoon into shallow bowls and serve with lemon wedges for squeezing over, if you like.

Soba noodle & edamame salad with grilled tofu

Ingredients

140g soba noodles

300g fresh or frozen podded edamame (soy) beans

4 spring onions, shredded

300g bag beansprouts

1 cucumber, peeled, halved lengthways, deseeded with a teaspoon and sliced

250g block firm tofu, patted dry and thickly sliced

1 tsp oil

handful coriander leaves, to serve

For the dressing

3 tbsp mirin

2 tsp tamari

2 tbsp orange juice

1 red chilli, deseeded, if you like, and finely chopped

Preparations

STEP 1

Heat dressing Ingredients in your smallest saucepan, simmer for 30 secs, then set aside.

STEP 2

Boil noodles following the pack instructions, adding the edamame beans for the final 2 mins cooking time. Rinse under very cold water, drain thoroughly and tip into a large bowl with the spring onions, beansprouts, cucumber, sesame oil and warm dressing. Season if you like.

STEP 3

Brush tofu with the veg oil, season and griddle or grill for 2-3 mins each side – the tofu is very delicate so turn carefully. Top the salad with the tofu, scatter with coriander and serve

Green bean & penne salad with tomato and olive dressing

Ingredients

75g wholemeal penne

160g green beans, trimmed and cut into short lengths

1 large red onion, halved and thinly sliced

2 tomatoes, chopped

1 tbsp rapeseed oil

2 tbsp apple cider vinegar

10g basil leaves

4 Kalamata olives, chopped

large handful rocket

Preparations

STEP 1

Boil the pasta in a pan of water for 5 mins. Add the beans and onion, return to the boil and cook for 5 mins more.

STEP 2

Meanwhile, put the tomatoes in a bowl with the oil, vinegar and basil (saving a couple of leaves), then blitz with a hand blender to make a dressing.

STEP 3

Drain the pasta and beans, tip into the dressing, add the olives and mix well. Spoon onto plates and top with the basil leaves and rocket, or pack into lunchboxes, cool, then top with the rocket and basil. Can be chilled for up to one day ahead.

Delicious End-of-the-week veggie noodles with ginger & tamari

Ingredients

1 nest wholewheat noodles (about 75g)

1 tbsp rapeseed oil

1 onion, halved and sliced

1 tbsp shredded ginger

2 garlic cloves, chopped

about 115g button mushrooms, quartered

about 65g Tenderstem broccoli, chopped

50g mixed nuts, roughly chopped

2 carrots, cut into noodles with a spiralizer or julienne peeler

1 tbsp tamari

⅓ small pack coriander, roughly chopped

Preparations

STEP 1

Pour boiling water over the noodles, leave them to soak for 5 mins, then drain.

STEP 2

Meanwhile, heat the oil in a wok and stir-fry the onion, ginger, garlic and mushrooms for 3-4 mins until starting to colour. Add the broccoli and nuts, and cook for a few mins more. Toss in the carrots and tamari, stir-fry until they just start to soften, then add the noodles and coriander.

Quinoa with stir-fried winter veg

Ingredients

200g quinoa

5 tbsp olive oil

2 garlic cloves, finely chopped

3 carrots, cut into thin sticks

300g leek, sliced

300g broccoli, cut into small florets

100g sundried tomato, drained and chopped

200ml vegetable stock

2 tsp tomato purée

juice 1 lemon

Preparations

STEP 1

Cook the quinoa according to pack instructions. Meanwhile, heat 3 tbsp of the oil in a wok or large pan, then add the garlic and quickly fry for 1 min. Throw in the carrots, leeks and broccoli, then stir-fry for 2 mins until everything is glistening.

STEP 2

Add the sundried tomatoes, mix together the stock and tomato purée, then add to the pan. Cover, then cook for 3 mins. Drain the quinoa, then toss in the remaining oil and the lemon juice. Divide between warm plates and spoon the vegetables on top.

Vegan paella

Ingredients

2 generous pinches of saffron

1 tbsp tomato purée

2 tsp vegetable bouillon powder

2 tbsp rapeseed oil

2 onions (320g), finely chopped

2 red peppers, deseeded and diced

3 garlic cloves, finely grated

2 tbsp soft thyme leaves

200g brown basmati rice

2 tsp smoked paprika

320g frozen broad beans

320g courgettes, halved and sliced

15g flat-leaf parsley, chopped

1 lemon, cut into wedges

Preparations

STEP 1

Put the kettle on to boil. Tip the saffron, tomato purée and bouillon powder into a large heatproof bowl, then pour over 1 litre boiling water and set aside.

STEP 2

Heat the oil in a large paella pan or frying pan over a medium heat and fry the onion for 5 mins, stirring often until starting to soften. Add the peppers, garlic and thyme, and cook for a few minutes more. Tip in the rice and paprika, and continue to cook, stirring for about a minute. Pour in the saffron stock, then cover and simmer for 10 mins.

Moroccan-style vegetable platter

Ingredients

2 tbsp rapeseed oil

2 garlic cloves, finely chopped

2 aubergines (about 500g), sliced

4 tomatoes, cut into wedges

1 tsp ground cumin

10g coriander, chopped

10g parsley, chopped

1 lemon, juiced

8 flatbreads

250g pack cooked beetroot, sliced

2 x 80g packs pomegranate seeds

1 mint sprig (optional)

For the dip

320g frozen baby broad beans

1 tsp cumin seeds

2 large garlic cloves

1 tbsp extra virgin olive oil

1 tsp smoked paprika

Preparations

STEP 1

For the dip, boil the broad beans for 7 mins, then drain, reserving the cooking water. Tip into a bowl with the cumin, garlic, oil, paprika and 6 tbsp of the reserved water, then blitz using a hand blender until smooth. Spoon into two small bowls.

STEP 2

Heat the oil in a pan over a medium heat and cook the garlic and aubergines, covered, for 10 mins, stirring occasionally until tender and slightly charred. Add the tomatoes and cumin, and cook for 5-10 mins, then turn off the heat. Add the herbs and lemon juice.

STEP 3

Serve half on a platter with one bowl of dip, four flatbreads and half the beetroot, along with the pomegranate seeds and mint, if using. You can warm the flatbreads in a frying pan or microwave before serving. Chill the remainder to eat cold the next day. Will keep covered and chilled for a day.

Vegan biryani

Ingredients

240g brown basmati rice

1½ tbsp rapeseed oil

1 large onion (220g), finely chopped

1 cinnamon stick

1 red chilli, deseeded and finely chopped (optional)

3 large garlic cloves, finely chopped

20g fresh ginger, peeled and finely chopped

1½ tsp cumin seeds

1 large red pepper, deseeded and roughly chopped

1 large aubergine (320g), cut into cubes

2 tbsp curry powder

400g can chopped tomatoes

2 tsp vegan bouillon powder

320g small cauliflower florets

30g coriander, stems and leaves separated and chopped

40g flame raisins

50g unsalted cashew nuts, toasted

Preparations

STEP 1

Rinse the rice until the water runs clear, then cook in a pan of fresh cold water following pack instructions for about 20 mins, or until almost tender.

STEP 2

Meanwhile, heat the oil in a large, deep frying pan over a medium heat and stir in the onion, cinnamon stick, chilli, garlic and ginger so they're coated in the oil. Scatter over the cumin seeds, cover and cook for 5 mins.

STEP 3

Stir well, then add the pepper and aubergine, and cook, stirring for 3-5 mins, until the veg is starting to soften. Stir in the curry powder, then the tomatoes and bouillon. Tip in the cauliflower florets, coriander stems and raisins, then cover and simmer for 10 mins over a medium-low heat.

Sticky noodles with homemade hoisin

Ingredients

For the hoisin

2 tbsp raisins

1 garlic clove

1 tbsp apple cider vinegar

2 tsp tomato purée

1 tsp tamari, plus extra to serve (optional)

1 tsp Chinese five spice

2 tbsp crunchy peanut butter (without palm oil or sugar)

For the stir-fry

2 nests wholemeal noodles (75g)

1 tsp rapeseed oil

1 tbsp chopped ginger

1 yellow pepper, deseeded and thinly sliced

2 red onions (173g), thinly sliced

100g long stem broccoli, halved

100g frozen soya beans, thawed

1 red chilli, seeded and chopped

handful basil leaves

Preparations

STEP 1

Put the raisins in a measuring jug or small, high-sided bowl, pour over 100ml boiling water then stir in the garlic, vinegar, tomato purée, tamari and five spice. Blitz with a hand blender until smooth, then stir in the peanut butter until well mixed.

STEP 2

Pour boiling water over the noodles and soak for 5 mins. Heat the oil in a non-stick wok, add the ginger with the vegetables and chilli and stir-fry for 5 mins or more until the veg have softened, but still have some bite.

Penne with cabbage & walnuts

Ingredients

400g wholemeal penne

3 tbsp rapeseed oil

500g savoy cabbage, shredded

2-3 chillies, deseeded and finely chopped

6 large garlic cloves, thinly sliced

30g walnuts (about 12 halves), chopped

½-1 lemon, zested and juiced

Preparations

STEP 1

Cook the penne in a pan of boiling water for 12 mins until tender. Meanwhile, heat the oil in a large pan over a medium heat and fry the cabbage for 8-10 mins until softened. Add the chilli and garlic and cook for 3-4 mins more until the garlic is starting to colour. Add the nuts and cook for 1 min more. Remove from the heat and stir in the lemon zest.

STEP 2

Drain the penne, reserving the cooking water. Add the drained pasta to the cabbage mixture along with the lemon juice and two ladlefuls of the reserved water (if needed, to loosen), and toss everything well to combine. Serve half between two people. Cool and chill the rest to eat another day. To serve, reheat in a pan over a low heat with a splash of water until piping hot – don't allow the penne to go soft. Will keep chilled for up to three days.

Courgette curry with lemon rice

Ingredients

For the curry

1 tbsp olive oil

2 tbsp ginger, very finely chopped

1½ tsp cumin seeds

1-2 red chillies, deseeded and finely chopped

6 garlic cloves, crushed

450g baby potatoes, thickly sliced

2 tsp ground coriander

1 tsp ground turmeric

4 large vine tomatoes, roughly chopped

1 tbsp tomato purée

200ml stock, made with 1 tsp vegetable bouillon powder

1 cinnamon stick

500g medium-sized courgettes, thickly sliced

15g chopped fresh coriander

For the lemon rice

1 tbsp olive oil

½-1 tsp brown mustard seeds (optional)

240g brown basmati rice

½-1 tsp turmeric

12 curry leaves (optional)

400g can chickpeas, drained

2 tbsp lemon juice

Preparations

STEP 1

Heat the oil in a large frying pan and fry the ginger for 3 mins. Stir in the cumin seeds, chillies and garlic and cook briefly, then add the potatoes, ground coriander and turmeric, and stir well. Tip in the tomatoes, tomato purée and stock, then add the cinnamon, cover, and leave to simmer for 5 mins.

STEP 2

Stir in the courgettes, then cover and cook for 10-12 mins until the courgettes are tender rather than soft. Stir in the fresh coriander.

STEP 3

Meanwhile, heat the oil in a pan and stir in the mustard seeds, if using, and cook until you hear them pop. Stir in the rice, turmeric and curry leaves, if using, then pour in 1 litre boiling water. Simmer, covered, for 15 mins, then add the chickpeas and lemon juice, cover once again, and cook for 10 mins more until the water has been absorbed and the rice is tender.

Mint & basil griddled peach salad

Ingredients

1 lime, zested and juiced

1 tbsp rapeseed oil

2 tbsp finely chopped mint, plus a few whole leaves to serve

2 tbsp basil, chopped

2 peaches (300g), quartered

75g quinoa

160g fine beans, trimmed and halved

1 small red onion, very finely chopped

1 large Little Gem lettuce (165g), roughly chopped

½ x 60g pack rocket

1 small avocado, stoned and sliced

Preparations

STEP 1

Mix the lime zest and juice, oil, mint and basil, then put half in a bowl with the peaches. Meanwhile, cook the quinoa following pack instructions.

STEP 2

Cook the beans for 3-4 mins until just tender. Meanwhile, griddle the peaches for 1 min on each side. If you don't have a griddle pan, use a large non-stick frying pan with a drop of oil.

STEP 3

Drain the quinoa and divide between shallow bowls. Toss the warm beans and onion in the remaining mint mixture and pile on top of the quinoa with the lettuce and rocket. Top with the avocado and peaches and scatter over the mint leaves. Serve while still warm.

Black bean chilli

Ingredients

2 tbsp olive oil

4 garlic cloves, finely chopped

2 large onions, chopped

3 tbsp sweet pimenton (Spanish paprika) or mild chilli powder

3 tbsp ground cumin

3 tbsp cider vinegar

2 tbsp brown sugar

2 x 400g (2 x 14oz) cans chopped tomatoes

2 x 400g (2 x 14oz) cans black beans, rinsed and drained

a few, or one, of the following to serve: crumbled feta cheese (or a dairy-free alternative), chopped spring onions, sliced radishes, avocado chunks, soured cream

Preparations

STEP 1

In a large pot, heat the olive oil and fry the garlic and onions for 5 mins until almost softened. Add the pimenton and cumin, cook for a few mins, then add the vinegar, sugar, tomatoes and some seasoning. Cook for 10 mins.

STEP 2

Pour in the beans and cook for another 10 mins. Serve with rice and the accompaniments of your choice in small bowls.

Lentil ragu with courgetti

Ingredients

2 tbsp rapeseed oil, plus 1 tsp

3 celery sticks, chopped

2 carrots, chopped

4 garlic cloves, chopped

2 onions, finely chopped

140g button mushrooms from a 280g pack, quartered

500g pack dried red lentils

500g pack passata

1l reduced-salt vegetable bouillon (we used Marigold)

1 tsp dried oregano

2 tbsp balsamic vinegar

1-2 large courgettes, cut into noodles with a spiraliser, julienne peeler or knife

Preparations

STEP 1

Heat the 2 tbsp oil in a large sauté pan. Add the celery, carrots, garlic and onions, and fry for 4-5 mins over a high heat to soften and start to colour. Add the mushrooms and fry for 2 mins more.

STEP 2

Stir in the lentils, passata, bouillon, oregano and balsamic vinegar. Cover the pan and leave to simmer for 30 mins until the lentils are tender and pulpy. Check occasionally and stir to make sure the mixture isn't sticking to the bottom of the pan; if it does, add a drop of water.

STEP 3

To serve, heat the remaining oil in a separate frying pan, add the courgette and stir-fry briefly to soften and warm through. Serve half the ragu with the courgetti and chill the rest to eat on another day. Can be frozen for up to 3 months.

Chickpea, tomato & spinach curry

Ingredients

1 onion, chopped

2 garlic cloves, chopped

3cm piece ginger, grated

6 ripe tomatoes

½ tbsp oil

1 tsp ground cumin

2 tsp ground coriander

1 tsp turmeric

pinch chilli flakes

1 tsp yeast extract (we used Marmite)

4 tbsp red lentils

6 tbsp coconut cream

1 head of broccoli, broken into small florets

400g can chickpeas, drained

100g bag baby spinach leaves

1 lemon, halved

1 tbsp toasted sesame seeds

1 tbsp chopped cashews, to mix with the sesame seeds

Preparations

STEP 1

Put the onion, garlic, ginger and tomatoes in a food processor or blender and whizz to a purée.

STEP 2

Heat oil in a large pan. Add the spices, fry for a few secs and add purée and yeast extract. Bubble together for 2 mins, then add lentils and coconut cream. Cook until lentils are tender, then add the broccoli and cook for 4 mins. Stir in chickpeas and spinach, squeeze over lemon and swirl through sesame and cashew mixture. Serve with brown rice, if you like.

Noodle salad with sesame dressing

Ingredients

For the dressing

1 tbsp sesame oil

2 tsp tamari

1 lemon, juiced

1 red chilli, deseeded and finely chopped

For the salad

1 small onion, finely chopped

2 wholemeal noodle nests (about 100g)

160g sugar snap peas

4 small clementines, peeled and chopped

160g shredded carrots

large handful of coriander, chopped

50g roasted unsalted cashews

Preparations

STEP 1

Mix all the dressing Ingredients together in a large bowl, then stir in the onion. Meanwhile, cook the noodles in a pan of boiling water for 5 mins, adding the sugar snap peas halfway through the cooking time – the noodles and peas should be just tender. Drain, cool under cold running water and drain again. Snip or cut the noodles into smaller lengths to make them more manageable to eat.

STEP 2

Tip the noodles and peas into the bowl with the dressing, along with the clementines, carrots, coriander and cashews. Toss to combine, then serve in bowls or pack into rigid airtight containers to take to work.

Carrot & pecan muffins

Ingredients

2 x 400g can cannellini beans in water, drained

2 tsp ground cinnamon

100g porridge oats

4 large eggs

2 tbsp rapeseed oil

4 tbsp maple syrup

2 tsp vanilla extract

zest 1 large orange

170g carrot, coarsely grated

100g raisins

80g pecan halves, 12 reserved, the rest roughly chopped

2 tsp baking powder

Preparations

STEP 1

Heat oven to 180C/160C fan/gas 4 and line a 12-hole muffin tin with paper cases. Tip the beans into a bowl and add the cinnamon, oats, eggs, oil, maple syrup, vanilla extract and orange zest. Blitz with a hand blender until really smooth – the beans and oats should be ground down as much as possible.

STEP 2

Stir in the carrot, raisins, chopped pecans and baking powder, and mix well. Spoon into the muffin cases – use a large ice cream scoop if you have one, to get nice even muffins.

STEP 3

Top each muffin with a reserved pecan and bake for 20 mins until set and light brown. Cool on a wire rack. Will keep in the fridge for a few days, or freeze for 6 weeks; thaw at room temperature

Instant berry banana slush

Ingredients

2 ripe bananas

200g frozen berry mix (blackberries, raspberries and currants)

Preparations

STEP 1

Slice the bananas into a bowl and add the frozen berry mix. Blitz with a stick blender to make a slushy ice and serve straight away in two glasses with spoons.

Crispy roasted chickpeas

Ingredients

1 x 400g can chickpeas, drained

1tsp rapeseed oil

2tsp smoked paprika

2tsp ground cumin

2tsp ground coriander

½tsp cayenne pepper

Preparations

STEP 1

Heat oven to 200C/180C fan/gas 4. Tip the chickpeas into a bowl and toss with the rapeseed oil, smoked paprika, cumin and coriander along with a big pinch of salt. Toss well until the chickpeas are well coated, then tip out onto a baking tray and bake for 35 mins, moving them round the tray halfway through so they dry out evenly and are crunchy. Leave to cool, then store in an airtight container.

Date & buckwheat granola with pecans & seeds

Ingredients

For the granola

85g buckwheat

4 medjool dates, stoned

1 tsp ground cinnamon

100g traditional oats

2 tsp rapeseed oil

25g sunflower seeds

25g pumpkin seeds

25g flaked almonds

50g pecan nuts, roughly broken into halves

50g sultanas (without added oil)

For the yogurt & fruit (to serve 2)

2 x 150ml pots low-fat bio natural yogurt

2 ripe nectarines or peaches, stoned and sliced

Preparations

STEP 1

Soak the buckwheat overnight in cold water. The next day, drain and rinse the buckwheat. Put the dates in a pan with 300ml water and the cinnamon, and blitz with a stick blender until completely smooth. Add the buckwheat, bring to the boil and cook, uncovered, for 5 mins until pulpy. Meanwhile, heat oven to 150C/130C fan/gas 2 and line two large baking trays with baking parchment.

STEP 2

Stir the oats and oil into the date and buckwheat mixture, then spoon small clusters of the mixture onto the baking trays. Bake for 15 mins, then carefully scrape the clusters from the parchment if they have stuck and turn before spreading out again. Return to the oven for another 15 mins, turning frequently, until firm and golden.

STEP 3

When the mix is dry enough, tip into a bowl, mix in the seeds and nuts with the sultanas and toss well. When cool, serve each person a generous handful with yogurt and fruit, and pack the excess into an airtight container. Will keep for a week. On other days you can vary the fruit or serve with milk or a dairy-free alternative instead of the yogurt.

Energy balls with dates

Ingredients

50g soft dried apricot

100g soft dried date

50g dried cherry

2 tsp coconut oil

1 tbsp toasted sesame seed

Preparations

STEP 1

Whizz apricots with dates and cherries in a food processor until very finely chopped. Tip into a bowl and use your hands to work in coconut oil.

Shape the mix into walnut-sized balls, then roll in sesame seeds. Store in an airtight container until you need a quick energy fix.

Avocado with tamari & ginger dressing

Ingredients

1small garlic clove, shredded

½ tsp shredded ginger

1 tsp tamari

2 tsp lemon juice

1 avocado

Preparations

STEP 1

Mix the garlic, ginger, tamari and lemon juice in a small bowl. Dilute with 1-2 tsp water. Cut the avocado in half and destone, then spoon in the dressing and eat with a teaspoon.

Polenta bruschetta with tapenade

Ingredients

700ml vegetable stock (Marigold Swiss vegetable bouillon is gluten and dairy-free)

140g instant polenta

2 tbsp chopped fresh basil

2 tbsp olive oil

9 tsp (about half a 190g jar) olive tapenade

9 SunBlush or semi-dried tomatoes, halved

100g mixed salad leaves

Preparations

STEP 1

Bring the stock to the boil in a saucepan, then reduce to a simmer. Stirring continuously, pour in the polenta in a steady steam and cook for 5 mins until thickened. Stir in the basil and season with black pepper and salt, if you like. Spread on an oiled shallow tin measuring 24 x 18cm. Leave to set for 1 hr.

STEP 2

Cut the polenta into 9 rectangles, each 8 x 6cm, then cut in half diagonally to make triangle shapes. Heat a griddle until hot, brush each triangle with oil and grill for 4-5 mins each side, until crisp and golden.

STEP 3

Top each triangle with 1/2 tsp tapenade and half a tomato. Serve warm on salad leaves.

Quinoa porridge

Ingredients

For the porridge (to serve 4)

175g quinoa

½ vanilla pod, split and seeds scraped out, or 0.5 tsp vanilla extract

15g creamed coconut

4 tbsp chia seeds

125g coconut yogurt

For the topping (to serve 2)

125g pot coconut yogurt

280g mixed summer berries, such as strawberries, raspberries and blueberries

2 tbsp flaked almonds (optional)

Preparations

STEP 1

Activate the quinoa by soaking overnight in cold water. The next day, drain and rinse the quinoa through a fine sieve (the grains are so small that they will wash through a coarse one).

STEP 2

Tip the quinoa into a pan and add the vanilla, creamed coconut and 600ml water. Cover the pan and simmer for 20 mins. Stir in the chia with another 300ml water and cook gently for 3 mins more. Stir in the pot of coconut yogurt. Spoon half the porridge into a bowl for another day. Will keep for 2 days covered in the fridge. Serve the remaining porridge topped with another pot of yogurt, the berries and almonds, if you like.

STEP 3

To have the porridge another day, tip into a pan and reheat gently, with milk or water. Top with fruit - for instance, orange slices and pomegranate seeds.

Vegetarian club

Ingredients

3 slices granary bread

1 large handful watercress

1 carrot, peeled and coarsely grated

small squeeze lemon juice

1 tbsp olive oil

2 dessertspoons reduced-fat hummus

2 tomatoes, thickly sliced

Preparations

STEP 1

Toast the bread. Meanwhile, mix the watercress, carrot, lemon juice and olive oil together. In a small bowl spread the hummus over each slice of toast. Top 1 slice with the watercress and carrot salad, sandwich with another slice of toast and top with the tomato. Lay the final slice of bread, hummus side down, then press down and eat as is or cut the sandwich into quarters.

Quinoa, peach & ginger bircher

Ingredients

200g quinoa

200g porridge oats

4 tsp finely grated ginger

225ml milk, plus a little extra if required

1 tbsp vanilla extract

6 x 120ml pots bio yogurt

6 ripe peaches

Preparations

STEP 1

Boil the quinoa in plenty of cold water for about 18 mins until the grains burst. Tip into a sieve and rinse under under cold water. Meanwhile, tip the oats into a large bowl with the ginger. Pour over 400ml boiling water and stir well. The mixture will become quite thick, but this process does stop the slightly starchy taste that some birchers made with cold water have. Stir in 225ml milk, the vanilla and

3 pots of yogurt, then fold through the quinoa. Cover and chill overnight.

STEP 2

The next day, add a little more milk to get the consistency you want, then spoon into six bowls. Top two with a ½ pot yogurt each and 2 stoned and chopped peaches, then mix together.

Avocado & strawberry ices

Ingredients

200g ripe strawberries, hulled and chopped

1 avocado, stoned, peeled and roughly chopped

2 tsp balsamic vinegar

½ tsp vanilla extract

1-2 tsp maple syrup (optional)

Preparations

STEP 1

Put the strawberries (save four pieces for the top), avocado, vinegar and vanilla in a bowl and blitz using a hand blender (or in a food processor) until as smooth as you can get it. Have a taste and only add the maple syrup if the strawberries are not sweet enough.

STEP 2

Pour into containers, add a strawberry to each, cover with cling film and freeze. Allow the pots to soften for 5-10 mins before eating.

Masala omelette muffins

Ingredients

olive oil, for greasing

2 medium courgettes, coarsely grated

6 large eggs

2 large or 4 small garlic cloves, finely grated

1 red chilli, deseeded and finely chopped

1 tsp chilli powder

1 tsp ground cumin

1 tsp ground coriander

handful fresh coriander, chopped

125g frozen peas

40g feta

Preparations

STEP 1

Heat oven to 220C/200C fan/ gas 7 and lightly oil four 200ml ramekins. Grate the courgettes and squeeze really well, removing as much liquid as possible. Put all the Ingredients except the feta in a large jug and mix really well.

STEP 2

Pour into the ramekins, scatter with the feta and bake on a baking sheet for 20-25 mins until risen and set. You can serve the muffins hot or cold with salad, slaw or cooked vegetables.

Red lentil & sweet potato pâté

Ingredients

1 tbsp olive oil, plus extra for drizzling

½ onion, finely chopped

1 tsp smoked paprika, plus a little extra

1 small sweet potato, peeled and diced

140g red lentil

3 thyme sprigs, leaves chopped, plus a little extra
to decorate (optional)

500ml low-sodium vegetable stock (choose a
vegan brand, if desired)

1 tsp red wine vinegar (choose a vegan brand, if
desired)

pitta bread and vegetable sticks, to serve

Preparations

STEP 1

Heat the oil in a large pan, add the onion and cook slowly until soft and golden. Tip in the paprika and cook for a further 2 mins, then add the sweet potato, lentils, thyme and stock. Bring to a simmer, then cook for 20 mins or until the potato and lentils are tender.

STEP 2

Add the vinegar and some seasoning, and roughly mash the mixture until you get a texture you like. Chill for 1 hr, then drizzle with olive oil, dust with the extra paprika and sprinkle with thyme sprigs, if you like. Serve with pitta bread and vegetable sticks.

Bean & feta spread with Greek salad salsa & oatcakes

Ingredients

400g can butter beans, drained

1 lemon, ½ juiced, ½ cut into 4 wedges

2 tbsp ricotta or bio yogurt

85g feta, crumbled

1 garlic clove

12 oatcakes

For the salsa

4 tomatoes, chopped

1 medium cucumber, finely diced

1 small red onion, finely chopped

12 pitted Kalamata olives, chopped

a few chopped mint leaves (optional)

Preparations

STEP 1

Tip the beans, lemon juice, ricotta, 50g feta and the garlic into a bowl and blitz with a hand blender or in a food processor to make a paste. Stir in the remaining feta and spoon the mixture into four small pots.

STEP 2

To make the salsa, stir all the Ingredients together with the mint (if using) and divide into four more pots, topping with a lemon wedge. These will keep, chilled in an airtight container, for two-three days. To eat, spread the oatcakes with the bean mixture, squeeze the lemon wedges over the salads and pile generously onto the oatcakes.

Melon & crunchy bran pots

Ingredients

½ x 200g pack melon medley

150g pot fat-free yogurt

2 tbsp fruit & fibre cereal

1 tbsp mixed seed

1 tsp clear honey

Preparations

STEP 1

Top melon medley with yogurt, then sprinkle over cereal mixed with seeds. Drizzle over honey and eat immediately.

Vegan kimchi

Ingredients

2-3 Chinese leaf (2kg prepared weight)

40-60g sea salt (3% of the cabbage weight)

1 tbsp seaweed (I use wakame), lightly rinsed

1 carrot

½ leek

2 spring onions

For the chilli paste

40g onion, chopped

40g garlic (10 cloves), peeled

5g ginger, chopped

1 small pear, cored and chopped

40g Korean chilli flakes (use less if you prefer it milder)

You will also need

a 2-litre sterilised jar

Preparations

STEP 1

Chop the Chinese leaf into bite-size pieces, weighing it until you have 2kg, then wash under running water. Mix the Chinese leaf with the salt and the seaweed in a large bowl. Set aside.

STEP 2

Every now and then, over the course of 3-4 hrs, mix the salted Chinese leaf and seaweed with your hands. (You will start to see liquid being released.) You want to be able to bend the Chinese leaf without breaking the pieces.

STEP 3

Meanwhile, shred the carrot and leek, and chop the spring onions. Set aside. Make the chilli paste by blitzing the onion, garlic, ginger and pear in a food processor until puréed. Add the chilli flakes, then blitz again to combine. Drain the Chinese leaf mixture, removing as much water as you can. This may take about 10 mins.

STEP 4

Toss the Chinese leaf mixture with the other vegetables, then mix in the chilli paste to coat everything. Tip into a 2-litre sterilised jar. Try not to have too many air pockets and leave a 1-inch space under the lid. Put a fermentation weight on top, or if you don't have one, try using some baking beans in a bag. Keep a plate under the jar in case of overflow. After 24-48 hrs you will begin to see bubbles appearing. That means fermentation is underway.

STEP 5

At any point during the fermentation, you can taste the kimchi to see how you like the flavour. I prefer to keep mine in the fridge after day 3 to slow down the process and start enjoying it. You can transfer the kimchi into smaller jars for easy access from the fridge. It also makes a great present for family and friends.

Chickpea, tomato & spinach curry

Ingredients

1 onion, chopped

2 garlic cloves, chopped

3cm piece ginger, grated

6 ripe tomatoes

½ tbsp oil

1 tsp ground cumin

2 tsp ground coriander

1 tsp turmeric

pinch chilli flakes

1 tsp yeast extract (we used Marmite)

4 tbsp red lentils

6 tbsp coconut cream

1 head of broccoli, broken into small florets

400g can chickpeas, drained

100g bag baby spinach leaves

1 lemon, halved

1 tbsp toasted sesame seeds

1 tbsp chopped cashews, to mix with the sesame seeds

Preparations

STEP 1

Put the onion, garlic, ginger and tomatoes in a food processor or blender and whizz to a purée.

STEP 2

Heat oil in a large pan. Add the spices, fry for a few secs and add purée and yeast extract. Bubble together for 2 mins, then add lentils and coconut cream. Cook until lentils are tender, then add the broccoli and cook for 4 mins. Stir in chickpeas and spinach, squeeze over lemon and swirl through sesame and cashew mixture. Serve with brown rice, if you like.

Red lentil & sweet potato pâté

Ingredients

1 tbsp olive oil, plus extra for drizzling

½ onion, finely chopped

1 tsp smoked paprika, plus a little extra

1 small sweet potato, peeled and diced

140g red lentil

3 thyme sprigs, leaves chopped, plus a little extra to decorate (optional)

500ml low-sodium vegetable stock (choose a vegan brand, if desired)

1 tsp red wine vinegar (choose a vegan brand, if desired)

pitta bread and vegetable sticks, to serve

Preparations

STEP 1

Heat the oil in a large pan, add the onion and cook slowly until soft and golden. Tip in the paprika and cook for a further 2 mins, then add the sweet potato, lentils, thyme and stock. Bring to a simmer, then cook for 20 mins or until the potato and lentils are tender.

STEP 2

Add the vinegar and some seasoning, and roughly mash the mixture until you get a texture you like. Chill for 1 hr, then drizzle with olive oil, dust with the extra paprika and sprinkle with thyme sprigs, if you like. Serve with pitta bread and vegetable sticks.

Griddled vegetables with melting aubergines

Ingredients

1 large aubergine

½a lemon, zested and juiced

3cloves of garlic, 1 crushed, 2 chopped

2 tbsp chopped parsley, plus extra to serve

1 tsp extra virgin olive oil, plus a little for drizzling

4 tsp omega seed mix (see tip)

2 tsp thyme leaves

1 tbsp rapeseed oil

1 red pepper, deseeded and cut into quarters

1 large onion, thickly sliced

2 courgettes, sliced on the angle

2 large tomatoes, each cut into 3 thick slices

8 Kalamata olives, halved

Preparations

STEP 1

Grill the aubergine, turning frequently, until soft all over and the skin is blistered, about 8-10 mins. Alternatively, if you have a gas hob, cook it directly over the flame. When it is cool enough to handle, remove the skin, finely chop the flesh and mix with the lemon juice, 1 chopped clove garlic, 1 tbsp parsley, 1 tsp extra virgin olive oil and the seeds. Mix the remaining parsley with the remaining chopped garlic and the lemon zest.

STEP 2

Meanwhile, mix the thyme, crushed garlic and rapeseed oil and toss with the vegetables, keeping the onions as slices rather than breaking up into rings. Heat a large griddle pan and char the vegetables until tender and marked with lines –

the tomatoes will need the least time. Pile onto plates with the aubergine purée and olives, drizzle over a little extra olive oil and scatter with the parsley, lemon zest and garlic.

Barbecue sesame sweet potatoes

Ingredients

6 sweet potatoes, washed and cut into wedges

3 tbsp vegetable oil

1 tsp toasted sesame oil

1 tbsp ginger, chopped

1 garlic clove, chopped

3 tbsp soy sauce

1 lime, juiced

1 tbsp sesame seeds (black if you have them)

50g plain peanuts, crushed

1 green chilli, sliced

½ bunch of spring onions, washed and chopped

Preparations

STEP 1

Light a lidded barbecue. Let the flames die down and the coals turn ashen, then mound the coal up on one side or heat an oven to 180C/160C fan/gas 4. Arrange the sweet potatoes on a large tray and drizzle with 1 tbsp of the vegetable oil, season and toss. Cook on the barbecue or in the oven for 25 mins until charred and softened.

STEP 2

Meanwhile, whisk the remaining oils, ginger, garlic, soy and lime juice. Baste the potatoes with some of the sauce and return to the barbecue for another 30-40 mins, basting as they cook. Once the potatoes are glazed and sticky, remove and sprinkle on the sesame seeds and peanuts, and leave to cool slightly. Remove the wedges from the tray and pop into a salad bowl. Sprinkle over the chilli and spring onions and serve.

Seeded soda bread

Ingredients

520g plain wholemeal flour, plus extra for dusting

50g four-seed mix (sunflower, pumpkin, sesame and golden flax seeds), plus extra for sprinkling

1½ tsp bicarbonate of soda

400ml fortified oat milk

2 tbsp lemon juice

Preparations

STEP 1

Heat the oven to 200C/180C fan/gas 6. Mix the flour, seeds and bicarb in a bowl, then mix together the milk and lemon juice in a small jug and pour it into the dry Ingredients. Stir with a knife until the mixture comes together into a sticky dough.

STEP 2

Tip onto a lightly floured work surface and lightly shape into a ball with wet or floured hands, as it will be sticky to handle. Lift onto a floured baking tray, reshape if required, then sprinkle more seeds over the top and press them in lightly. Bake for 35-40 mins until firm and golden. Cool on a wire rack, then wrap in foil until needed. Will keep chilled for up to four days, or frozen for up to a month.

Red cabbage with apples

Ingredients

1 red cabbage, finely shredded

2 bay leaves

5 star anise

½ tsp ground cinnamon

200ml vegetable stock or water

50g golden caster sugar

75ml cider vinegar

2 apples, cored and cut into wedges

Preparations

STEP 1

Place all the Ingredients except for the apples in a large saucepan and season. Place over a medium heat, bring to the boil, then turn down the heat and simmer for 30 mins. Add the apples, then continue cooking for 15 mins until tender.

Pickled red cabbage

Ingredients

500g red cabbage, finely shredded

1tbsp coarse sea salt

500ml cider vinegar

200ml red wine

300-400g granulated sugar

2tsp black peppercorn

6 bay leaves

2tbsp yellow mustard seed

Preparations

STEP 1

Place the shredded cabbage in a colander over the sink and sprinkle with salt. Leave for 2-3 hours, then drain and wash away the salt. Pay dry with a clean tea towel.

STEP 2

Put the vinegar, wine, sugar (300g if you prefer a sharper flavour or 400g for a sweeter taste), peppercorns and bay leaves into a big, wide saucepan and simmer until the liquid has reduced by about half. Set aside for 10 mins to infuse.

STEP 3

Strain through a fine sieve into a jug or bowl, and discard the peppercorns and bay leaves. Put the cabbage and mustard seeds into a big bowl, and then pour the strained liquid over. Transfer the cabbage and pickling liquid into sterilised jars and seal. Will last for a month in the fridge.

Spiced apple crisps

Ingredients

2 Granny Smiths

cinnamon, for sprinkling

Preparations

STEP 1

Heat the oven to 160C/ 140C fan/ gas mark 3. Core the apple and slice through the equator into very thin slices 1 - 2mm thick. Dust with cinnamon and lay flat on a baking sheet lined with parchment paper.

STEP 2

Cook for 45 mins – 1 hour, turning halfway through and removing any crisps that have turned brown. Continue cooking until the apples have dried out and are light golden. Cool, store in an airtight container and enjoy as a snack.

Summer sautéed potatoes

Ingredients

1 ½kg potato, cut into small chunks

4 tbsp rapeseed oil

1 tbsp butter

4 bay leaves

2 garlic cloves (don't worry about peeling)

zest 1 lemon

small bunch parsley, chopped

Preparations

STEP 1

Place the potatoes in a large pan, cover with water and bring to the boil. Simmer for 5-8 mins until starting to soften but not falling apart. Drain and leave to steam-dry in the colander for a few mins.

STEP 2

Heat the oil and butter in a large frying pan. Scrunch up the bay leaves in your hands and add them to the pan along with the whole garlic cloves. Once the potatoes are dry, tip into the pan and season. Toss them in the pan and cook over a medium-high heat for 20-25 mins, turning often, using a fish slice so you don't break them up.

STEP 3

When the potatoes are crisp and golden, grate the lemon zest straight over and cook for 1-2 mins more. Taste for seasoning, then scatter with parsley and serve.

Thai carrot & radish salad

Ingredients

4 tbsp sweet chilli dipping sauce

zest 1 lime and 2 tbsp juice

1 tsp fish sauce

1 Little Gem lettuce, separated into leaves

2 carrots, cut into thin batons

10 radishes, sliced

4 spring onions, cut on the diagonal

handful roughly chopped coriander

Preparations

STEP 1

Mix the chilli sauce with the lime zest and juice, and fish sauce to make the dressing.

STEP 2

Arrange the lettuce in a large salad bowl. Toss all the remaining Ingredients with the dressing just before you are ready to eat, to keep everything crisp and fresh, then add to the lettuce.

Red cabbage with mulled Port & pears

Ingredients

1 large red cabbage, quartered, cored and thinly sliced

1 large onion, sliced

200ml port

1 large cinnamon stick

pinch ground cloves

2 star anise

2 tbsp soft brown sugar

1 tbsp red wine vinegar

4 pears, diced

Preparations

STEP 1

Put all the Ingredients except the pears in a large pan and cover with a tight- fitting lid. Cook on a low heat for 1 hr, then stir through the pears. Cover and cook for 1 hr more until the cabbage is really tender. If at any point the cabbage looks dry, add a splash of water. If there is still liquid in the pan at the end, turn the heat right up to evaporate it. Season with a little salt and serve. The cabbage can be prepared ahead and either chilled or frozen. Then reheat in the pan or in a microwave.

Carrot & sugar snap salad

Ingredients

1 tbsp hoisin sauce

juice ½ lime

2cm/¾in fresh ginger, peeled and grated

200g sugar snap peas, thinly sliced

3 carrots, coarsely grated

½ small bunch coriander, roughly chopped

Preparations

STEP 1

Make the dressing by whisking the hoisin, lime juice and ginger with 2 tbsp cold water.

STEP 2

In a large bowl, mix the sugar snap peas, carrots and coriander. Pour over the dressing and mix to coat.

CHAPTER 9
Health Benefits and Considerations

In 2015, the School of Public Health at the University of Memphis released findings from a study investigating the anti-inflammatory and anti-cancer potential of macrobiotic diets. The study compared the nutrient composition of a macrobiotic diet plan compared to national dietary recommendations (RDA) based on the National Health and Nutrition Examination Survey (NHANES).

A key comparison was assessing which approach scored high on the dietary inflammatory index (DII), in addition to comparing levels of total calories, macronutrients and 28 micronutrients.

Findings showed that the macrobiotic diet plan had a lower percentage of energy from fat, higher intake of dietary fiber and higher amounts of most micronutrients. Nutrients in the macrobiotic diet often met or exceeded RDA recommendations, with the exception of vitamin D, vitamin B12 and calcium.

Based on DII scores, the macrobiotic diet was found to be "more anti-inflammatory compared to NHANES data," and the researchers concluded that overall findings indicated potential for disease prevention when following a macrobiotic eating approach.

2. May Help Improve Heart Health

Certain studies have found evidence for macrobiotic-style diets supporting cardiovascular health — in particular lowering serum lipid levels and lowering blood pressure levels. This isn't surprising considering how many high-antioxidant, anti-inflammatory foods are encouraged in a macrobiotic diet.

For example, the macrobiotic diet is rich in dietary fiber, including all sorts of high-fiber foods, such as veggies, beans and unprocessed ancient grains. Eating plenty of fiber has been correlated with improvements in cardiovascular disease risk factors through multiple mechanisms, including lipid reduction, body weight regulation, improved glucose metabolism, blood pressure control and reduction of chronic inflammation.

3. Can Help Support a Healthy Weight and Relationship to Eating

Much like those eating the Okinawa way, proponents of the macrobiotic diet focus not only on eating the right foods, but also eating them in the right amounts. Eating mindfully, slowing down and savoring meals, paying attention to physical sensations (also called biofeedback), and thoroughly chewing food are all emphasized in the macrobiotic diet.

This approach can help you better manage how much you eat, give you more enjoyment from having less, teach you to avoid emotional eating out of boredom or other negative feelings, and achieve satiety more easily. Rather than trying to lose weight just by eliminating many foods or consuming less, which can lead you to feel overly hungry and deprived, eating mindfully and choosing foods wisely can help you feel more in touch with your body's needs.

4. Very Low in Sugar, Gluten and Packaged Foods

Like other whole food-based diets that eliminate junk foods, packaged products, bottled drinks, fried foods and fast foods, the macrobiotic diet is very low in sugar, empty calories and artificial ingredients. This makes it a very nutrient-dense diet, high in things like vitamin C, vitamin E and fiber but overall low in calories.

It can also be potentially beneficial for those with food allergies since it eliminates common allergens that can cause indigestion, such as dairy products, almost all gluten and nightshades. However, one drawback and point of critique is that macrobiotic diets tend to include lots of salty, high-sodium foods, mostly from things like soy sauce, fermented soy products and sea veggies.

5. May Be Able to Help Prevent Cancer

Although diet is only one piece of the total puzzle when it comes to preventing cancer, and results vary from person to person, research suggests that consuming a macrobiotic diet can help lower the risk for cancer partly by providing high levels of antioxidants and phytoestrogens.

A 2011 report published in the Journal of Nutrition stated, "On the basis of available evidence and its similarity to dietary recommendations for chronic disease prevention, the macrobiotic diet probably carries a reduced cancer risk." Women consuming macrobiotic diets tend to have modestly lower circulating estrogen levels, which has been tied to a lowered risk of breast cancer.

Macrobiotic diets provide high amounts of phytoestrogens from foods like fermented soy products and sesame seeds, and these may help regulate production of natural estrogen by binding to estrogen receptor sites. While too much estrogen comes with its own risks, in the case of women over the age of 50 who naturally experience decreased levels during menopause, extra estrogen from their diets might help decrease cancer risk, among other benefits.

www.ingramcontent.com/pod-product-compliance
Lightning Source LLC
Chambersburg PA
CBHW051739250726
48659CB00001B/140